Kidney Diet Cookbook for Seniors

25 Easy & Delicious Recipes to Prevent Chronic Kidney Disease

By Dr. Amelia Wellness

FREE BONUS

14 Day Meal Plan added at the end of the recipes book. Feel free to modify quantities and snacks based on personal preferences and dietary requirements. This meal plan offers a variety of flavors while promoting renal health in older people. Consult a healthcare expert for personalized guidance

TABLE OF CONTENT

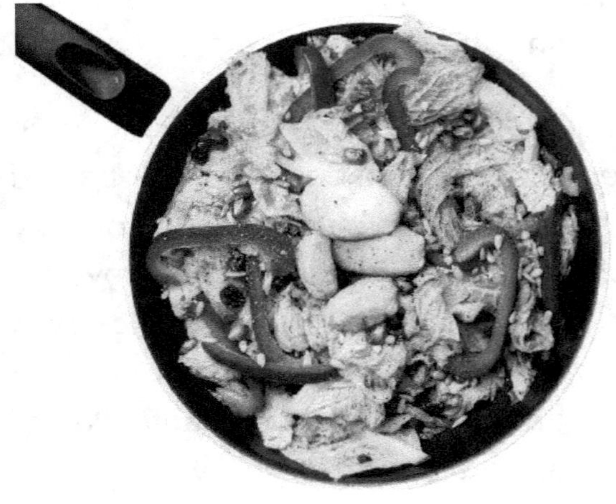

Introduction

In "Delicious Recipes to Prevent Chronic Kidney Disease for Old People," we go on a culinary adventure with Kelvin, a tenacious guy determined to manage and prevent chronic kidney disease in his golden years. Kelvin's experience is motivating because it demonstrates how making conscious and mindful nutritional choices may have a big impact on kidney health.

Kelvin found consolation and empowerment in the pages of this cookbook as he battled chronic renal disease. With a collection of tasty dishes for seniors, he acquired a new love for the combination of flavorful cuisine with kidney-friendly components. Kelvin's journey exemplifies the transformational potential of conscious eating, as he not only avoids further deterioration but also adopts a lifestyle that promotes total well-being.

This cookbook becomes Kelvin's valued companion, providing him with a broad selection of recipes that not only tantalise the taste senses but also address the nutritional requirements necessary for kidney health. From rich stews to vibrant salads, each dish is carefully created to find a balance between flavour and nutrition. As Kelvin embarks on his culinary expedition, readers are invited to join him on a journey of renewal, demonstrating that the kitchen may actually be a haven for health and longevity.

25 EASY & DELICIOUS RECIPES

Grilled Lemon Herb Salmon

Ingredients:

- Salmon filets

- Lemon juice

- Fresh herbs (rosemary, thyme)

- Olive oil.

Instructions:

1. Marinate salmon in lemon juice, herbs, and olive oil.

2. Grill until fully done.

Quinoa and Vegetable Stir-Fry

Ingredients:

- Quinoa - Mixed vegetables (bell peppers, broccoli, carrots) - Low-sodium soy sauce.

- Sesame oil

Instructions:

1. Cook quinoa.

2. Cook vegetables and mix with soy sauce and sesame oil.

Cauliflower and Chickpea Curry

Ingredients:

- Cauliflower - Chickpeas.
- Coconut Milk
- Curry Spices

Instructions:

1. Cook cauliflower with chickpeas in coconut milk with curry spices.

Mediterranean Chickpea Salad

Ingredients:

- Chickpeas - Cherry tomatoes.

- Cucumber

- Feta Cheese

- Olive Oil

Instructions:

1. Combine the chickpeas, tomatoes, cucumber, and feta.

2. Drizzle with olive oil

Baked Herb Chicken

Ingredients:

- Chicken breasts

- Garlic Powder

- Italian herbs.

- Olive Oil

Instructions:

1. Season chicken with garlic powder and Italian herbs.

2. Finish with a drizzle of olive oil.

Spinach and Mushroom Omelette

Ingredients:

- Eggs.

- Spinach

- Mushrooms.

Instructions:

3. Use low-sodium cheese. - To prepare, whisk eggs, then add spinach, mushrooms, and cheese.

4. Cook like an omelette

Roasted Vegetable Skewers

Ingredients:

- Bell peppers

- Zucchini

- Cherry tomatoes.

- Olive Oil

Instructions:

5. Thread vegetables on skewers.

6. Roast with a little layer of olive oil.

Sweet Potato and Black Bean Chili

Ingredients:

- Sweet potatoes

- Black bean

- Tomatoes

- Chilli spices.

Instructions:

7. Mix sweet potatoes, black beans, tomatoes, and chilli seasonings.

8. Simmer until the flavours blend.

Lemon Garlic Shrimp

Ingredients:

- Shrimp

- Lemon

- Garlic

- Fresh parsley

Instructions:

To prepare, sauté prawns with lemon, garlic and parsley.

Brown Rice Pilaf

Ingredients:

- Brown rice

- Onion - Peas

- Low-sodium vegetable broth

Instructions:

9. Saute onion, then add brown rice and peas, cook with vegetable broth.

Caprese Salad with Balsamic Glaze

Ingredients:

- Tomatoes

- Fresh mozzarella

- Basil leaves

- Balsamic glaze.

Instructions:

10. Arrange tomato, mozzarella, and basil.

11. Drizzle with balsamic glaze.

Grilled Eggplant Parmesan

Ingredients:

- Eggplant slices

- Marinara sauce.

- Parmesan cheese

- Olive oil

Instructions:

12. Grill eggplant, cover with marinara and Parmesan, and bake until bubbling.

Lentil and Vegetable Soup

Ingredients:

- Lentils

- Carrots

Instructions:

13. Cook lentils, carrots, and celery in low-sodium broth.

Turkey and Vegetable Kabobs

Ingredients:

- Turkey breast

- Bell peppers

- Red onions

- Olive Oil

Instructions:

14. Skewer the turkey and veggies.

15. Grill with a bit of olive oil

Greek Yoghurt Parfait

Ingredients:

- Greek yoghurt.

- Berries

- Granola

- Honey

Instructions:

16. Prepare by layering Greek yoghurt, berries, and granola.

17. Drizzle with honey.

Pesto Zoodles

Ingredients:

- Zucchini noodles

- Cherry tomatoes

- Pesto sauce

- Pine nuts

Instructions:

18. Toss zoodles and tomatoes with pesto.

19. Garnish with pine nuts.

Broccoli and Almond Stir-Fry

Ingredients:

- Broccoli
- Almonds
- Soy sauce
- Ginger

Instructions:

20. Stir-fry broccoli and almonds with soy sauce and ginger.

Berry Spinach Smoothie

Ingredients:

- Spinach

- Mixed berries

- Greek yogurt

- Almond milk

Instructions:

21. Blend spinach, berries, yogurt, and almond milk.

Baked Cod with Herbs

Ingredients:

- Cod fillets

- Dill

- Lemon zest

- Olive oil

Instructions:

22. Season cod with dill and lemon zest.

23. Bake with a drizzle of olive oil.

Asparagus and Tomato Frittata

Ingredients:

- Asparagus

- Cherry tomatoes

- Eggs

- Parmesan cheese

Instructions:

24. Saute asparagus and tomatoes, pour beaten eggs over.

25. Bake until set, sprinkle with Parmesan.

Chickpea and Spinach Stew

Ingredients:

Chickpeas

- Spinach
- Tomatoes
- Cumin

- Vegetable broth

Instructions:

To prepare, simmer chickpeas, spinach, tomatoes, cumin, and vegetable broth.

Salmon and Dill Avocado Salad

Ingredients:

- Smoked salmon

- Avocado.

- Fresh dill

- Mixed greens.

Instructions:

Prepare by arranging smoked salmon, avocado, and mixed greens.

Garnish with fresh dill

Vegetable and Lentil Casserole

Ingredients:

- Lentils.

- Bell peppers with carrots

- Tomato Sauce

Instructions:

Mix lentils, bell peppers, carrots, and tomato sauce.

Bake until the vegetables are soft.

Turkey and Sweet Potato Hash

Ingredients:

- Ground turkey
- Sweet potatoes.
- Onion
- Paprika.

Instructions:

26. Brown turkey with sweet potatoes, onion, and paprika.

Cucumber and Mint Infused Water

Ingredients:

- Cucumber slices

- Fresh mint leaves.

- Water.

Instructions:

Mix cucumber slices with mint leaves in water.

Allow to infuse for a refreshing hydration.

14 DAYS MEAL PLAN

Here's a 14-day meal plan to guide you

Day 1:

- Breakfast: Greek Yogurt Parfait

- Lunch: Quinoa and Vegetable Stir-Fry

- Dinner: Grilled Lemon Herb Salmon with Roasted Vegetable Skewers

 Day 2:

- Breakfast: Berry Spinach Smoothie

- Lunch: Lentil and Vegetable Soup

- Dinner: Cauliflower and Chickpea Curry with Brown Rice Pilaf

 Day 3:

- Breakfast: Pesto Zoodles

- Lunch: Turkey and Vegetable Kabobs

- Dinner: Mediterranean Chickpea Salad with Baked Cod with Herbs

Day 4:
- Breakfast: Vegetable and Lentil Casserole
- Lunch: Chickpea and Spinach Stew
- Dinner: Asparagus and Tomato Frittata

Day 5:
- Breakfast: Lemon Garlic Shrimp
- Lunch: Broccoli and Almond Stir-Fry
- Dinner: Salmon and Dill Avocado Salad

Day 6:
- Breakfast: Cucumber and Mint Infused Water
- Lunch: Sweet Potato and Black Bean Chili
- Dinner: Grilled Eggplant Parmesan

Day 7:
- Breakfast: Caprese Salad with Balsamic Glaze

- Lunch: Baked Herb Chicken
- Dinner: Spinach and Mushroom Omelette

Day 8:
- Breakfast: Berry Spinach Smoothie
- Lunch: Quinoa and Vegetable Stir-Fry
- Dinner: Grilled Lemon Herb Salmon with Roasted Vegetable Skewers

Day 9:
- Breakfast: Pesto Zoodles
- Lunch: Lentil and Vegetable Soup
- Dinner: Cauliflower and Chickpea Curry with Brown Rice Pilaf

Day 10   :
- Breakfast: Cucumber and Mint Infused Water
- Lunch: Mediterranean Chickpea Salad
- Dinner: Baked Cod with Herbs and Greek Yogurt Parfait

Day 11:
- Breakfast: Vegetable and Lentil Casserole
- Lunch: Chickpea and Spinach Stew
- Dinner: Asparagus and Tomato Frittata

Day 12:
- Breakfast: Lemon Garlic Shrimp
- Lunch: Broccoli and Almond Stir-Fry
- Dinner: Salmon and Dill Avocado Salad

Day 13:
- Breakfast: Caprese Salad with Balsamic Glaze
- Lunch: Baked Herb Chicken
- Dinner: Spinach and Mushroom Omelette

Day 14:

- Breakfast: Sweet Potato and Black Bean Chili
- Lunch: Turkey and Sweet Potato Hash
- Dinner: Grilled Eggplant Parmesan

Feel free to modify quantities and snacks based on personal preferences and dietary requirements. This meal plan offers a variety of flavours while promoting renal health in older people. Consult a healthcare expert for personalised guidance.

9 798877 814844